STUDIES IN CHARACTER

Twelve Transformational Studies of the Character That Makes for Character Healthy Living

Dr. Stephen & Megan Scheibner

Character Health Corporation
CARY, NORTH CAROLINA

Studies in Character
Twelve Transformational Studies of the Character That Makes for Character Healthy Living

By Dr. Stephen and Megan Scheibner
Copyright © 2014. All rights reserved.

Produced and Distributed by:

Character Health Corporation
101 Casablanca Ct.
Cary, NC 27519

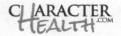

CharacterHealth.com

ISBN: 978-0-9849714-4-2

Printed in the United States

Dedication

To all our faithful supporters who read our
character quality emails each week...

This book is our gift to you.

Don't grow weary of doing well!

Contents

HOW TO USE THIS STUDY

As with any Bible study, the more effort you put into the study... the more benefit you'll receive from the study! Studies in Character is designed to challenge and encourage your walk with the Lord, without frustrating you by making the study so difficult that it is a burden, or so simple that it seems like "busy work". Our goal was to strike a nice balance! For those of you who desire to go deeper, look in the back of the study! There you'll find ideas to provide extra opportunities for growth through scripture look-ups and memorization.

Each lesson of the study combines short-answer questions and thought-provoking quotes from famous people. Some of the people quoted are Christians, while some are not. Take your time and really consider what is stated in the quotations. As believers, we must train our minds to recognize truth and to discard untruth, or in some cases, "false" truth. Read the quotes prayerfully with an eye to discern when something "sounds right," but in reality, is not aligned with Scripture.

For the short-answer questions, please answer each question thoroughly. One-word or overly simplistic answers may fulfill the "check in the block," requirement of completing the study, but you will miss the opportunity to reap deep spiritual growth.

At the back of each chapter, you will find a goal page intended to be used as you write three personal goals related to the study. Set practical, yet challenging goals to help you incorporate and build into your life the character quality that you just finished studying. Without a plan, change will not happen! We would encourage you to share your goals with a trusted friend and ask them to hold you accountable to reaching those goals.

Our prayer is that Studies in Character will challenge and equip you to live a courageous, Christlike, and character-healthy life... A life that honors and glorifies God and reaches others with the Gospel of Christ.

God Bless,
Steve and Megan

Integrity

DEFINITION: Firm adherence to a code of moral or artistic values. Incorruptibility.

To be known as a man or a woman of integrity should be the goal of every follower of Christ. Integrity goes far beyond what the world sees, and encompasses who we are in our innermost being. A simple measure of the quality of your integrity is this: whom you are when no one is looking. A true man or woman of integrity seeks to be righteous in his words, actions, and even thought life, at all times, regardless of the presence or lack of an audience.

To have integrity means to be complete. A ship will not be launched into the sea until it has integrity. In other words, the whole thing must hold together without leaking. Psalm 41:12 translates the Hebrew word Tom to the English word integrity.

Tom means; completeness, fullness, wholeness, perfection, soundness or integrity. If you think of a life characterized by integrity you are really thinking about a life that will hold together under adverse temptation or pressure. Proverbs 2:7 reminds us that God will be a shield to those who have integrity... those who don't "cave-in" when the pressure to compromise comes their way.

The Greek language of the New Testament provides even more insight into the importance of integrity. James 1:4 translates the Greek word *Holokleros* to the English word *Perfect* or *Complete*. Perfect here does not mean sinless perfection rather it means integrity. *Holokleros* means to be whole, having all of its parts to be sound or perfect.

Holokleros is actually two words put together as one.

Holo means; All the whole

Kleros means; A part or share

Holokleros means that which retains all, which it was allotted to it at first wanting nothing for its completeness, bodily, mentally or morally.

Like the perfection of man before the fall, the *Holokleros* is one who has preserved, or having once lost has now regained his completeness.

For the believer, we can only regain completeness through Christ. We cannot have integrity apart from a relationship with Christ and we cannot have integrity if we allow compromise or worldliness in any area of our lives. To accept such concession in even one part of our lives is to have no integrity.

Let's look at the life of Esther as an excellent example of one who has integrity.

1. Read Esther 4:10-17. Did Esther have any guarantee that the King would welcome her into his presence? What gave Esther the courage to align herself with her people, the Jews? Explain.

   _____

   _____

   _____

   _____

_____

_____

_____

_____

_____

_____

_____

2. Read I Kings 9:3-5. In verse 4, what does integrity of the heart and uprightness look like? (Hint, finish the verse to find the answer)
   Write out your answer below...

_____

_____

_____

_____

_____

_____

_____

_____

_____

_____

_____

_____

_____

In what areas of life is God calling you to walk more in integrity and uprightness today? Make a list...

_____

_____

_____

_____

_____

_____

_____

_____

_____

_____

_____

3. Read I Chronicles 29:17. Because David was a man of integrity, he could have no fear when God did what? Write out your answer.

_____

_____

_____

_____

_____

_____

_____

_____

_____

Is this your daily desire to stand fearless as God tries your heart?

_____

_____

_____

_____

William Clement
_____
Stone: (4 May 1902–3
_____
September 2002) was
_____
an American business-
man, author, and philan-
_____
thropist; an advocate of
_____
what he called **"PMA"**:
_____
Positive Mental Attitude.
_____
Beginning with meager
material resources he
_____
became a multi-million-
_____
aire, was nominated for
the Nobel Peace Prize,
_____
and lived to be 100.

_____

_____

_____

_____

"Have the courage to say no. Have the courage to face the truth. Do the right thing because it is right. These are the magic eyes to living your life with integrity."

—W. Clement Stone

Do you agree or disagree with the quote by Stone?
Write out your thoughts…

_____

_____

_____

_____

_____

_____

_____

_____

_____

_____

_____

_____

_____

_____

_____

_____

_____

_____

5. Read Psalms 25:21 and Proverbs 13:6. What benefit will integrity provide for you? There is no guarantee that mud won't be thrown at you. However, if you are a man or woman of integrity — It Won't Stick!! Write out your answer below.

6. In Psalms 78:72 we are told that David shepherded his people according to the integrity of his heart. Practically speaking, how would you define integrity of heart? Explain your answer in the space provided.

7. Read Proverbs 10:9 and 11:3. What will integrity of the heart provide in our walk with the Lord? Explain your answer.

_____

_____

_____

_____

_____

_____

_____

_____

_____

_____

_____

8. Although Abraham provides many examples of faithful obedience to the Lord, in the area of integrity he made several serious mistakes. Read Genesis 12:9-13. Why did Abram ask Sarai to lie? Write out your answer.

_____

_____

_____

_____

_____

_____

_____

_____

_____

_____

_____

_____

_____

_____

9. Although our families may have long-term issues that demonstrate a lack of integrity, this is no reason for us to portray the same issues. Ask the Lord to show you where you lack integrity, then confess, repent, and move on.

10. Although God will always be delighted with our integrity of heart, the world and other believers may not always be so thrilled. Read Proverbs 29:10. In this verse, blameless may also be translated, "of integrity." Bear up under evil reactions; nothing in this world makes giving up your integrity a worthwhile action!

"Integrity is what we do, what we say, and what we say we do."

—Don Galer

Integrity

List 3 goals for personal growth in the character quality of Integrity...

1) _____

_____

_____

_____

_____

_____

2) _____

_____

_____

_____

_____

_____

3) _____

_____

_____

_____

_____

_____

Personal Notes on Integrity

_____

_____

_____

_____

_____

_____

_____

_____

_____

_____

_____

_____

_____

_____

_____

_____

_____

_____

_____

_____

_____

_____

Diligence

DEFINITION: persevering application; the attention or care legally required of a person.

D iligence is the difference between a job simply finished and a job well done. All areas of a believer's life should be approached with diligence and such diligence will draw attention *to* and increase our testimony *for* Christ.

1. Read Ruth 2:5-12. How did Boaz characterize Ruth's sacrifices?
   Write out your answer.

   _____

   _____

   _____

   _____

   _____

   What blessing did he pray for her? List the blessings.

   _____

   _____

   _____

_____

_____

_____

2. What does Proverbs 10:4 say that diligent hands will bring about?

_____

_____

_____

_____

_____

_____

_____

_____

3. Read Proverbs 12:24. What will the diligent hand do? Explain your answer.

_____

_____

_____

_____

_____

_____

_____

_____

Diligence

How do you see Proverbs 12:24 in action in daily life?
Write your answer.

_____

_____

_____

_____

_____

_____

_____

_____

_____

_____

_____

_____

_____

_____

_____

_____

"Being forced to work, and forced to do your best, will breed in you temperance and self-control, diligence and strength of will cheerfulness and content, and a hundred virtues which the idle will never know."

—Charles Kingsley

Charles Kingsley (June 12, 1819 – January 23, 1875) was an English novelist, particularly associated with the West Country and north-east Hampshire. In addition to his literary body of work, Kingsley was a Protestant priest, who gained prominence in the public arena as an activist for politics and social reform. His commitment to his social agenda manifested itself in his written work, not only in his many published letters, sermons, scientific essays, and lectures, but also as themes in his novels and historical works.
His notoriety gained him a professorship at Cambridge University, and the canon at Westminster. He was also chaplain to Queen Victoria and tutor to the future King Edward VII.

4. React to the quote above. Do you agree or disagree? Write out your answer.

_____

_____

_____

_____

_____

_____

_____

_____

_____

5. The NASB translates Proverbs 12:27 this way, "A slothful man does not roast his prey, but the precious possession of a man is diligence." Restate this Proverb in your own words.

_____

_____

_____

_____

_____

_____

_____

_____

_____

6. Read Proverbs 13:4. What does it mean that the soul of the diligent is made fat? Write out your answer below.

_____

_____

_____

_____

_____

_____

_____

_____

_____

_____

7. The opposite of diligence is laziness. Titus 1:12 portrays the testimony of a certain group of people. What is said of the Cretans?

_____

_____

_____

_____

_____

_____

_____

_____

_____

Search your heart and ask a friend, what would be said of you? Are you diligent or lazy? Record what you discover.

_____

_____

_____

_____

_____

_____

_____

_____

_____

8. Finally, read I Timothy 4:13-15. In what areas was Timothy to show special diligence? Explain your answer.

_____

_____

_____

_____

_____

_____

_____

_____

_____

Diligence

"Few things are impossible to diligence
and skill."

—Samuel Johnson

27

List 3 goals for personal growth in the character quality of Diligence...

1) _____

_____

_____

_____

_____

_____

2) _____

_____

_____

_____

_____

_____

3) _____

_____

_____

_____

_____

_____

Personal Notes on Diligence

_____

_____

_____

_____

_____

_____

_____

_____

_____

_____

_____

_____

_____

_____

_____

_____

_____

_____

_____

_____

_____

_____

_____

_____

Honesty

DEFINITION: A fairness and straight forward-
ness of conduct; adherence to the facts.

**Job 6:25a says, "How painful are honest
words!"**

The Hebrew word *Yosher* is translated honest in Job 6:25.
Yosher means straightness, right, equity, uprightness,
truth, duty or honesty. Such honesty directs good people
in right paths.

*In other words, straight talk is our duty. Telling the truth is
not optional rather it is the right thing for honest upright
children of God to do! Painful or not, we must always
tell the truth.*

Honesty is a character quality that by it's very definition has
very little wiggle room. Either you are known to be honest or you
are not. Either you can be trusted to tell the truth, both in words
and actions, or you cannot. A reputation for being dishonest is
not easily changed or overcome, so let's allow scripture to mold
our character of honesty.

1. Read Luke 8:41-47. We know that Jesus knew all things and
    could have immediately identified who had touched Him.

The woman, however, did not know that. She would have assumed that she could have denied touching Jesus with no one to prove otherwise. Her response to Jesus' questions shows her character of honesty.

Is Honesty as important when it is probable that you won't get caught? Write out your answer.

_____

_____

_____

_____

_____

_____

Can you share a time when you were honest, even when no one would have known if you weren't? Record your answer below.

_____

_____

_____

_____

_____

_____

_____

What was the end result of your honesty?

_____

_____

_____

_____

_____

_____

_____

_____

2. Another word for dishonesty is the word guile. Read John 1:47 and record the high praise Jesus gave one of his future disciples. Can people say the same about you? Yes or No?

_____

_____

_____

_____

_____

_____

_____

_____

_____

_____

_____

3. Read II Kings 12:11-15. Why was there no accounting required? Write out your answer below.

_____

_____

Mary Kay Ash (May 12, 1918 – November 22, 2001) was an American businesswoman and founder of *Mary Kay Cosmetics, Inc.* Ash was widely respected. She considered the Golden Rule the founding principle of Mary Kay Cosmetics, and the company's marketing plan was designed to allow women to advance by helping others to succeed. She advocated "praising people to success" and her slogan "God first, family second, career third" expressed her insistence that the women in her company keep their lives in balance.

Notice how these men's character preceded them!

"Honesty is the cornerstone of all success, without which confidence and ability to perform shall cease to exist."

—**Mary Kay Ash**

React to this quote. Do you agree or disagree?

_____

_____

_____

_____

_____

_____

_____

_____

_____

_____

4. Read Leviticus 19:35-36. Honesty is not simply what we say, but our actions, as well. How were the people to show their character of honesty?

_____

_____

_____

_____

_____

_____

_____

_____

_____

_____

_____

_____

In what ways can we show "just balances" today?

_____

_____

_____

_____

_____

_____

_____

_____

_____

_____

5. In 1 Chronicles 29:17, the word uprightness can also be translated as honest intent. When God tries our hearts and evaluates our sacrifices to Him, what is He hoping to find?

_____

_____

_____

_____

_____

_____

_____

_____

_____

_____

6. Job 6:25a says this: "How painful are honest words." Sometimes, being honest with a friend may bring momentary
   pain into our lives. However, read Proverbs 27:6 to see the
   good result of those painful honest words. What is that
   good result?

_____

_____

_____

_____

_____

_____

_____

_____

_____

_____

7. Sometimes, no one knows we have been dishonest, but in our
   heart, we know. Read Matthew 26:69-75. Did anyone know
   that Peter had been dishonest as he denied his relationship
   with Christ? Explain your answer.

_____

_____

_____

_____

_____

_____

_____

_____

_____

_____

How did Peter respond to his own dishonesty?

_____

_____

_____

_____

_____

_____

_____

8. Read Ephesians 4:25-27. According to this scripture, who is exempt from honesty?

_____

_____

_____

_____

_____

_____

_____

When we are dishonest, to whom are we opening the door, thereby allowing access into our lives and relationships?

_____

_____

_____

_____

_____

_____

_____

_____

_____

_____

_____

"Honesty is the best policy. If I lose mine honor, I lose myself." —William Shakespeare

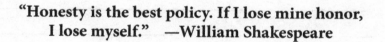

William Shakespeare

(baptised 26 April 1564; died 23 April 1616) was an English poet and playwright, widely regarded as the greatest writer in the English language and the world's pre-eminent dramatist. He is often called England's national poet and the "Bard of Avon". His surviving works, including some collaborations, consist of about 38 plays, 154 sonnets, two long narrative poems, and several other poems. His plays have been translated into every major living language and are performed more often than those of any other playwright.

List 3 specific goals for personal growth in the character quality of Honesty...

1) _____

_____

_____

_____

_____

_____

_____

2) _____

_____

_____

_____

_____

_____

3) _____

_____

_____

_____

_____

_____

Personal Notes on Honesty

Respect

DEFINITION: High and special regard; to consider worthy of high regard.

Romans 12:17 says, "Never pay back evil for evil to anyone. Respect what is right in the sight of all men."

The Greek word for respect means to think beforehand, to provide for, to take thought of or be careful of beforehand. Respect therefore, is something that is assigned in advance.

Respect is not something assigned at the moment based upon how you feel rather it is something established ahead of time based on well-established norms.

Respect is an almost forgotten character quality. Instructions such as, "Respect your elders" and "Be respectful" have virtually disappeared from our conversations. Even the dictionary definition seems to make respect optional, contingent on whether we consider a person or object to be worthy of our respect. However, how should a Christian live? Let's consider scripture and some biblical characters to determine the value of respect in our lives.

1. Read I Samuel 24:3-7. When we read this account, Saul had been pursuing David without cause, seeking to kill him. David would have been justified in killing Saul to protect himself. Why then does verse 5 say that David's conscience bothered him?
Explain your answer below.

_____

_____

_____

_____

_____

_____

_____

_____

_____

_____

_____

Saul's life was spared because David understood respect for the Lord's anointed.

2. Who are some of the people in your life to whom God wants you to show respect? List some by name.

_____

_____

_____

_____

_____

When we show respect for these people, regardless of whether or not they are respected by others, our testimony as a follower of Christ is strengthened.

3. Read Leviticus 19:3 and 19:32. To which two groups are we instructed to show respect? How can you show that respect in a practical daily way? Explain...

_____

_____

_____

_____

_____

_____

_____

"Respect for ourselves guides our morals; respect for others guides our manners."

—Laurence Sterne

Laurence Sterne (24 November 1713–18 March 1768) was an Irish novelist and an Anglican clergyman. He is best known for his novels *The Life and Opinions of Tristram Shandy, Gentleman*, and *A Sentimental Journey Through France and Italy*; but he also published many sermons, wrote memoirs, and was involved in local politics. Sterne died in London after years of fighting consumption.

React to the quote above, do you agree or disagree?

_____

_____

_____

_____

_____

_____

_____

_____

3. Proverbs 11:16 instructs us to evaluate what type of woman gains respect.

Ladies: What practical things are you doing to develop this reputation? Write your answer below.

_____

_____

_____

_____

_____

_____

_____

_____

Gentlemen: What things do you notice in a young woman's life that you would see as kind-hearted? Write your answer below.

_____

_____

_____

_____

_____

_____

_____

_____

5. In I Peter 2:17, the word honor can also be translated respect. Who does this verse command us to respect? Does the verse indicate that they must earn our respect?

_____

_____

_____

_____

_____

_____

_____

_____

_____

6. In I Samuel 23:4-7, we read that David respected Saul's position and spared his life. In contrast, Saul's life ended when a young man did not understand the value of this type of respect, resulting in Saul's death and disastrous consequences for the young man, himself.

    Read II Samuel 1:1-16. Did the young man think he was doing a good or bad thing?

    _____

    _____

    _____

    _____

    _____

    _____

    Why did David deal so harshly with his actions?

    _____

    _____

    _____

    _____

    _____

7. Too many times, as we follow the crowd in showing disrespect to those in authority over us, we put to death our own testimony. We lead others into harmful disrespect and kill our opportunity to show others the difference Christ has made in our lives.

Can you think of a time that your lack of respect led a younger brother or sister in Christ to go even further down the road of disrespect? What were the consequences of your poor example?

_____

_____

_____

_____

_____

_____

_____

_____

_____

8. Recognizing that, as believers we are all slaves of the Lord Jesus Christ will help us to render respect with the right attitude.

Read Ephesians 6:5-6. From where should our respect for others emanate? List...

_____

_____

_____

_____

_____

_____

9. Read Hebrews 10:24. As we extend respect to others, whether they seem to deserve it or not, we encourage both the one being respected and those around us. Can you remember a time that your heartfelt respect was an encouragement to someone else?

_____

_____

_____

_____

_____

_____

_____

_____

_____

_____

_____

_____

"Respect yourself if you would have
others respect you."
—Baltasar Gracian

Baltasar Gracián y Morales, SJ
(January 8, 1601 – December 6, 1658) was a Spanish Jesuit and baroque prose writer. He was born
in Belmonte, near Calatayud (Aragon). The son of a
doctor, in his childhood Gracián lived with his uncle,
who was a priest. He studied at a Jesuit school in
1621 and 1623 and theology in Zaragoza. He was
ordained in 1627 and took his final vows in 1635.
He assumed the vows of the Jesuits in 1633 and
dedicated himself to teaching in various Jesuit schools. He spent time in Huesca, where he
befriended the local scholar Vincencio Juan de
Lastanosa, who helped him achieve an important
milestone in his intellectual upbringing. He acquired
fame as a preacher, although some of his oratorical
displays, such as reading a letter sent from Hell from
the pulpit, were frowned upon by his superiors. He
was named Rector of the Jesuit college of Tarra-
gona and wrote works proposing models for courtly
conduct such as *El héroe* (The Hero), *El político* (The
Politician), and *El discreto* (The Discreet One). During
the Spanish war with Catalonia and France, he was
chaplain of the army that liberated Lleida in 1646.

List 3 specific goals for personal growth in the character quality of Respect...

1) _____

_____

_____

_____

_____

2) _____

_____

_____

_____

_____

3) _____

_____

_____

_____

_____

_____

Respect

Personal Notes on Respect

Thankfulness

DEFINITION: Express gratitude to; say thanks; hold responsible. Grateful; appreciative.

---

1 Corinthians 1:4 states, "I thank my God always concerning you, for the grace of God which was given you in Christ Jesus."

The Greek word translated thanks is Eucharisteo from which we get the word Eucharist. It means to be thankful, to thank, to speak well of or to eulogize.

Being thankful costs us nothing and yet on a daily basis we too often hold on stingily to the words or actions of thankfulness. As forgiven believers, our thankful attitudes should overflow and set us apart as a grateful people.

Are you grateful for Christ's substitutionary death on the cross for you?

1. Read Luke 17:11-19. How many lepers were healed?

_____

_____

_____

_____

How many lepers displayed thankfulness? Write out your answer.

_____

_____

_____

_____

_____

_____

_____

From verse 18, what did the one leper's thankfulness give to God? Explain.

_____

_____

_____

_____

_____

2. Read Hebrews 12:28. When we are thankful, what do we offer to God? Explain below.

_____

_____

_____

_____

_____

_____

_____

_____

_____

_____

_____

By contrast, what do you think a lack of thankfulness says about our God?

_____

_____

_____

_____

_____

_____

_____

_____

_____

_____

_____

_____

_____

_____

4. In Psalms 50:23, how do we honor God? List the ways.

_____

_____

_____

_____

_____

_____

_____

_____

_____

_____

_____

_____

_____

_____

_____

_____

_____

_____

_____

_____

_____

_____

_____

_____

"All of our discontents about what we want appear to spring from the want of thankfulness for what we have."   —Daniel Defoe

---

Daniel Defoe (ca. 1659-1661–24 April 1731), born Daniel Foe, was an English writer, journalist, and pamphleteer, who gained enduring fame for his novel *Robinson Crusoe*. Defoe is notable for being one of the earliest proponents of the novel, as he helped to popularize the form in Britain, and is even referred to by some as among the founders of the English novel. A prolific and versatile writer, he wrote more than 500 books, pamphlets, and journals on various topics (including politics, crime, religion, marriage, psychology and the supernatural). He was also a pioneer of economic journalism.

React to this quote. Do you agree or disagree?

_____

_____

_____

_____

_____

_____

_____

_____

_____

_____

_____

_____

5. Read Psalms 69:30, 95:2, and 147:7. What activity is linked with the giving of thanks? Explain your answer.

_____

_____

_____

_____

_____

_____

_____

_____

_____

Does thankfulness characterize your participation in this activity?

_____

_____

_____

_____

_____

_____

_____

_____

_____

_____

6. In I Corinthians 1:4-5, for what did Paul always thank God? Make a list below.

_____

_____

_____

_____

_____

_____

_____

_____

_____

Is there someone in your life that evokes this kind of thanksgiving in your heart? Have you told them?

_____

_____

_____

_____

_____

_____

_____

_____

_____

_____

7. Turn back to Luke 17:16. The healed leper did not just thank Jesus, he was exuberant in his thanks! How did he show this exuberant thankfulness? Explain.

_____

_____

_____

_____

_____

_____

_____

_____

How can you show exuberant thankfulness in your life? List the ways.

_____

_____

_____

_____

_____

_____

_____

_____

_____

_____

8. Read Philippians 4:6. What should accompany our prayers and requests? Write out your answer.

_____

_____

_____

_____

_____

_____

_____

_____

_____

How will remembering this change our approach to prayer? Explain your answer.

_____

_____

_____

_____

_____

_____

_____

_____

9. 1 Thessalonians 5:18 tells us what things in our lives should cause us to express thankfulness. What are those things?

_____

_____

_____

_____

_____

_____

10. There is no end to the things for which we can be thankful. Begin a list today of the things, both large and small, for which you are thankful. Train yourself to thank God with an overflowing, exuberant thankfulness. What's on your list!!

_____

_____

_____

_____

_____

> **"One of life's gifts is that each one of us,
> no matter how tired and downtrodden,
> finds reason for thankfulness: for the crops
> carried in from the fields and the grapes
> from the vineyard."**
>
> —J. Robert Moskin

Thankfulness

List 3 specific goals for personal growth in the character quality of Thankfulness...

1) _____

_____

_____

_____

_____

_____

2) _____

_____

_____

_____

_____

3) _____

_____

_____

_____

_____

_____

_____

Personal Notes on Thankfulness

Generosity

DEFINITION: the quality or fact of being characterized by a noble or forbearing spirit; magnanimous, forbearing, kindly.

God wants us to be generous, not envious! An overflowing, abundantly generous believer gives off the scent of their Lord Jesus Christ. Let's examine scripture to build our understanding of this Godly character quality.

1. Read Acts 9:36. Dorcas was not simply known because of her deeds of kindness and charity; she was known for how she practiced those deeds. How was it that she practiced her deeds of kindness? Make a list below.

_____

_____

_____

_____

_____

_____

_____

_____

_____

Generosity is not once and done, it is a continual overflowing of good deeds!

2. Generosity does not depend on our own financial situation. Read II Corinthians 8:1-2. Although the churches in Macedonia were suffering great poverty, what was their response to other believer's needs? Write out your answer.

_____

_____

_____

_____

_____

_____

_____

_____

_____

_____

_____

_____

_____

_____

_____

3. In II Corinthians 9:11, as Paul exhorted the Corinthians to liberality or generosity, what did he tell them that their liberality would produce? Explain.

_____

_____

_____

_____

_____

_____

_____

_____

As the Corinthians gave, God would be thanked. Does your generous life lead others in thanksgiving to God? Yes or No? Explain your answer...

_____

_____

_____

_____

_____

_____

_____

_____

_____

_____

_____

"He who gives what he would as readily throw away gives without generosity; for the essence of generosity is in self sacrifice."

—Henry Taylor

Sir Henry Taylor (18 October 1800 – 27 March 1886) was an English dramatist. Taylor was born in Bishop Middleham, the son of a gentleman farmer, and spent his youth in Witton-le-Wear with his stepmother at Witton Hall (now Witton Tower) in the high street. His father George was a friend of Wordsworth and the poet visited him in July 1838.

In Witton, Taylor wrote 'The Cave of Ceada' which was accepted for the *Quarterly Review*. He became editor of the *London Magazine* in 1823, and from 1824 until 1872, he worked in the Colonial Office. Taylor wrote a number of plays, including *Isaac Comnenus* (1827) and *Philip van Artevelde* (1834). This latter brought him fame and elicited comparisons with Shakespeare In 1845 there followed a book of lyrical poems. His essay 'The Statesman' (1836) caused some controversy, being a satirical view of how the civil service really works. Taylor published his Autobiography in 1885, which contains pleasant portraits of Wordsworth, Southey, Tennyson and Scott among others.

Do you agree or disagree with this quote?

_____

_____

_____

_____

_____

_____

4. Read Psalms 37:23-26. The psalmist describes the steps of the man God delights in, how is that man characterized in verse 26? Give details.

_____

_____

_____

_____

_____

_____

_____

_____

_____

_____

5. Proverbs 11:25 and 22:9 show us the fruit of generosity. What is that fruit?

_____

_____

_____

_____

_____

_____

_____

_____

6. The opposite of generosity is stinginess, an unwillingness to share what we have. In Mark 10:13, with whom were the disciples unwilling to share the Lord Jesus, resulting in a rebuke from their Lord? Write out your answer.

_____

_____

_____

_____

_____

_____

_____

_____

_____

_____

7. From I Timothy 6:18, how would you define generosity?

_____

_____

_____

_____

_____

_____

_____

_____

_____

_____

8. Read Matthew 20:1-15. Why were the first workers so upset? Explain your answer.

_____

_____

_____

_____

_____

_____

_____

_____

_____

_____

Do you find yourself upset when others receive something you think you deserve? Yes or No? Why or why not?

_____

_____

_____

_____

_____

_____

_____

_____

_____

_____

_____

With what word is that attitude described in verse 15?

_____

_____

_____

_____

_____

_____

_____

_____

_____

_____

_____

9. Finally, in II Corinthians 9:6, we see the comparison between giving and receiving. Restate this verse in your own words. Write your answer below.

_____

_____

_____

_____

_____

_____

_____

_____

_____

_____

_____

_____

"Children should be taught not the little virtues, but the great ones. Not thrift, but generosity and an indifference to money; not caution but courage and a contempt for danger; not a desire for success, but a desire to be and to know."

—Natalia Ginzburg

Natalia Ginzburg née Levi (July 14, 1916, Palermo—October 7, 1991, Rome) was an Italian author whose work explored family relationships, politics, and philosophy.

List 3 specific goals for personal growth in the character quality of Generosity...

1) _____

_____

_____

_____

_____

_____

2) _____

_____

_____

_____

_____

3) _____

_____

_____

_____

_____

_____

_____

Personal Notes on Generosity

_____

_____

_____

_____

_____

_____

_____

_____

_____

_____

_____

_____

_____

_____

_____

_____

_____

_____

_____

_____

_____

_____

_____

_____

Patience

DEFINITION: The capacity, habit, or fact of bearing pains or trial calmly without complaint. Manifesting forbearance under provocation or strain, steadfast, not hasty or impetuous.

The Greek word that often translates patience is the word *Hupomeno*, which means to remain under. It means to have patience toward things and circumstances especially in the midst of adversity.

*Patience sometimes seems such an unattainable character quality that it becomes easier to joke about it, rather than buckle down and develop patience. Quips such as, "Sorry I must have prayed for patience," or "I'd never have the patience for **that!**" remind us that the only way to develop patience is through the hard work of trials and repetition. Let's not avoid the hard work, but rather allow God's Word to shape our view of patience.*

1. The opposite of patience is impatience, not wanting to wait, wanting to act, or even more often, speak, when the timing is not right. Read Esther 5:1-8 and Esther 7:1-10, to see how Esther's patience paved the way for the Jew's lives to be spared.

    Write any insights you gain below.

_____

_____

_____

_____

_____

_____

_____

_____

_____

_____

2. Patience is sometimes translated *forbearance*. Read Proverbs 25:15 to see the principle Esther practiced in Esther chapters 5 and 7. What principle is this? Write out your answer.

_____

_____

_____

_____

_____

_____

_____

_____

_____

_____

3. Another word translated patience is the word *discretion*. In Proverbs 19:11, what will a man's patience make him slow to do? Explain.

_____

_____

_____

_____

_____

_____

_____

Do you see this principle in your own life? Yes or no? Why or why not?

_____

_____

_____

_____

_____

_____

_____

_____

_____

_____

"A man who is a master of patience is master of everything else." —George Savile

George Savile, 1st
Marquess of Halifax PC
(11 November 1633–5
April 1695) was an
English statesman, writer,
and politician.

React to this quote. Do you agree or disagree?

_____

_____

_____

_____

_____

_____

4. Read Ecclesiastes 7:8. With what is patience contrasted?

_____

_____

_____

_____

_____

_____

_____

How do you see that contrast evident in your daily life? Give details.

_____

_____

_____

_____

_____

_____

_____

_____

_____

5. In Romans 2:4, we see the end result of God's kindness, for-bearance, and patience. What is that end result? Write out your answer.

_____

_____

_____

_____

What heart attitude should this invoke in believers?

_____

_____

_____

_____

_____

6. Read Colossians 1:9-12. Patience joins other character qualities in Paul's prayer for the Colossians. What are all of the character qualities that Paul prayed the Colossian believers would attain? List them below.

_____

_____

_____

_____

_____

_____

_____

_____

_____

_____

_____

_____

_____

Is that your prayer for your own life today? Why or Why not?

_____

_____

_____

_____

_____

7. Although Rebecca knew that God had a plan for her son, Jacob, she was impatient to see it carried out. Read Genesis 27:1-13 and 41-45. What was the final result of her impatience?

_____

_____

_____

_____

_____

_____

_____

_____

_____

Rebecca never saw her precious Jacob again. Too often, the easy impatient choice leads to awful lifelong consequences. Can you think of any easy choices you have made that left you with unpleasant long-term consequences?

_____

_____

_____

_____

_____

_____

_____

8. One area we need to show especial patience is in our handling of the Word of God. Read II Timothy 4:2. What are we to do with great patience and instruction?
   Write out your answer.

_____

_____

_____

_____

_____

_____

_____

9. Jesus Christ is our perfect example. How is His patience characterized in I Timothy 1:16? Explain your answer.

_____

_____

_____

_____

_____

_____

_____

_____

_____

_____

"We ought to give thanks for all fortune: if it is good, because it is good, if bad, because it works in us patience, humility and the contempt of this world and the hope of our eternal country."

—C.S. Lewis

Clive Staples Lewis (29 November 1898 – 22 November 1963), commonly referred to as C. S. Lewis and known to his friends and family as Jack, was an Irish-born British novelist, academic, medievalist, literary critic, essayist, lay theologian and Christian apologist. He is also known for his fiction, especially *The Screwtape Letters, The Chronicles of Narnia* and *The Space Trilogy.*

Lewis was a close friend of J. R. R. Tolkien, and both authors were leading figures in the English faculty at Oxford University and in the informal Oxford literary group known as the "Inklings". According to his memoir *Surprised by Joy*, Lewis had been baptised in the Church of Ireland at birth, but fell away from his faith during his adolescence. Owing to the influence of Tolkien and other friends, at the age of 32 Lewis returned to Christianity, becoming "a very ordinary layman of the Church of England". His conversion had a profound effect on his work, and his wartime radio broadcasts on the subject of Christianity brought him wide acclaim.

In 1956, he married the American writer Joy Gresham, 17 years his junior, who died four years later of cancer at the age of 45. Lewis died three years after his wife, as the result of renal failure. His death came one week before his 65th birthday. Media coverage of his death was minimal, as he died on 22 November 1963 —the same day that U.S. President John F. Kennedy was assassinated, and the same day another famous author died, Aldous Huxley.

Lewis's works have been translated into more than 30 languages and have sold millions of copies. The books that make up The Chronicles of Narnia have sold the most and have been popularized on stage, TV, radio and cinema.

List 3 specific goals for personal growth in the character quality of Patience...

1) _____

_____

_____

_____

_____

2) _____

_____

_____

_____

_____

3) _____

_____

_____

_____

_____

_____

Patience

Personal Notes on Patience

_____

_____

_____

_____

_____

_____

_____

_____

_____

_____

_____

_____

_____

_____

_____

_____

_____

_____

_____

_____

_____

Responsibility

DEFINITION: The quality or state of being liable to be called to account as the primary cause, motive, or agent, able to answer for one's conduct and obligations.

R esponsibility is a character quality that sets apart mature believers

All believers are called to be obedient, but responsible believers go beyond simple obedience to what they are commanded, to an awareness of what is needed and a commitment to fulfill those needs.

1. Read I Samuel 17:23-26 and 32-37. How did a young shepherd take responsibility to protect the reputation of God?

_____

_____

_____

_____

_____

_____

2. In Matthew 27:3-4 and 24-25, responsibility is translated "see to it yourself." What responsibilities were Judas and Pilate trying to shirk?

_____

_____

_____

_____

_____

_____

_____

_____

_____

_____

3. Read Acts 6:1-4. What responsibility did the disciples need to delegate?

_____

_____

_____

_____

_____

_____

_____

_____

What were the disciple's primary responsibilities to encompass?

_____

_____

_____

_____

_____

_____

_____

_____

_____

_____

4. In Acts 6, the disciples wisely delegated responsibilities in order to be able to fulfill their own responsibilities. What happens when we refuse to delegate responsibilities or we take on more responsibilities than we can handle?

_____

_____

_____

_____

_____

_____

_____

"Responsibility is the price of greatness."
—Winston Churchill

Sir Winston Leonard Spencer-Churchill, (30 November 1874 – 24 January 1965) was a British politician and statesman known for his leadership of the United Kingdom during the Second World War (WWII). He is widely regarded as one of the great wartime leaders. He served as prime minister twice (1940–1945 and 1951–1955). A noted statesman and orator, Churchill was also an officer in the British Army, a historian, writer, and an artist. To date, he is the only British prime minister to have received the Nobel Prize in Literature, and the first person to be recognised as an honorary citizen of the United States.

During his army career, Churchill saw military action in India, the Sudan and the Second Boer War. He gained fame and notoriety as a war correspondent and through contemporary books he wrote describing the campaigns. He also served briefly in the British Army on the Western Front in the First World War (WWI), commanding the 6th Battalion of the Royal Scots Fusiliers.

At the forefront of the political scene for almost fifty years, he held many political and cabinet positions. Before WWI, he served as President of the Board of Trade, Home Secretary and First Lord of the Admiralty as part of the Asquith Liberal government. During the war, he continued as First Lord of the Admiralty until the disastrous Gallipoli Campaign caused his departure from government. He returned as Minister of Munitions, Secretary of State for War, and Secretary of State for Air. In the interwar years, he served as Chancellor of the Exchequer in the Conservative government.

After the outbreak of the WWII, Churchill was again appointed First Lord of the Admiralty. Following the resignation of Neville Chamberlain on 10 May 1940, he became Prime Minister of the United Kingdom and led Britain to victory against the Axis powers. Churchill was always noted for his speeches, which became a great inspiration to the British people, as well as to the embattled Allied forces.

After the Conservative Party lost the 1945 election, he became Leader of the Opposition. In 1951, he again became Prime Minister, before retiring in 1955. Upon his death, the Queen granted him the honour of a state funeral, which saw one of the largest assemblies of statesmen in the world.

React to the quote by Churchill. Do you agree or disagree?

_____

_____

_____

_____

_____

_____

_____

_____

5. Read Acts 18:4-6. For what did Paul claim no responsibility?

_____

_____

_____

_____

_____

Why? Explain your answer.

_____

_____

_____

_____

_____

_____

6. In II Chronicles 31:11-21, we see that Hezekiah faithfully appointed responsibilities to the Levites, who in turn were faithful to fulfill those responsibilities. Read verse 18 and record how the Levites embraced their responsibilities.

_____

_____

_____

_____

_____

_____

_____

_____

_____

_____

7. II Chronicles 31:20-21 reveals Hezekiah's heart attitude regarding his own responsibilities to the Lord. What was that attitude? Write our your answer.

_____

_____

_____

_____

_____

_____

_____

_____

8. Early in Genesis, we see a different attitude toward responsibility. Read Genesis 4:8-10. How did Cain approach his responsibility to his brother's well being? Give details.

_____

_____

_____

_____

_____

_____

_____

_____

_____

9. Can you think of areas in your own life that your attitude is like Cain's, echoing "Am I my brother's keeper?" What do you think God's response would be?

_____

_____

_____

_____

_____

_____

_____

_____

"We are in a fight for our principles and
our first responsibility is to live by them."

—President George W. Bush

George Walker Bush (born July 6, 1946, in
New Haven, Connecticut) was the 43rd President of the United States, serving from 2001 to
2009, and the 46th Governor of Texas, serving
from 1995 to 2000.

Responsibility

List 3 specific goals for personal growth in the character quality of Responsibility...

1) _____

_____

_____

_____

_____

_____

2) _____

_____

_____

_____

_____

_____

3) _____

_____

_____

_____

_____

_____

_____

Personal Notes on Responsibility

Joy

DEFINITION: The emotion evoked by wellbeing, success, or good fortune or by the process of possessing what one desires, delight, a source or cause of great delight.

If, as the dictionary definition states, joy is the process of possessing what one desires, we Christians have the greatest cause for joy.

We possess joy not just for the present only, but for eternity. As you would expect, scripture has much to say about the topic of joy.

1. Read Acts 3:1-9. What reaction of joy did the lame man show in verse 8?

2. In verse 9-10 of Acts 3, we see the domino effect of joy. What did the lame man's joy evoke in the people who observed his behavior?

_____

_____

_____

_____

_____

_____

_____

_____

3. Read Nehemiah 8:10. What is the source of our strength? Explain your answer.

_____

_____

_____

_____

_____

_____

_____

_____

_____

"I certainly wasn't happy. Happiness has to do with reason, and only reason earns it. What I was given was the thing you can't earn and can't keep, and often don't even recognize at the time; I mean joy."

—Ursula K. LeGuin

React to this quote. Do you agree or disagree?

Ursula Kroeber Le Guin (Born October 21, 1929) is an American author. She has written novels, poetry, children's books, essays, and short stories, most notably in the genres of fantasy and science fiction. First published in the 1960s, her works explore Taoist, anarchist, ethnographic, feminist, psychological and sociological themes.

4. In Job 6:10, why did Job rejoice in spite of unsparing pain? Write out your answer.

_____

_____

_____

_____

_____

_____

_____

How can you rejoice in spite of pain and trials in your life? Give details.

_____

_____

_____

_____

_____

_____

_____

_____

_____

_____

_____

5. Read I Thessalonians 1:6. Although the Thessalonians received the Word with much tribulation, where did they still find their joy?

_____

_____

_____

_____

_____

_____

_____

_____

6. Read John 16:24. What will make our joy complete? List your answer below.

_____

_____

_____

_____

_____

_____

_____

_____

7. A lack of joy causes bitterness in our hearts. After the repentance of Ninevah, Jonah's reaction should have been joy and thankfulness. Instead, he succumbed to bitterness. Read Jonah 3:10-4:1. What sin accompanied Jonah's bitterness?

_____

_____

_____

_____

_____

_____

_____

8. Read Romans 12:12. In what should we rejoice? Explain below.

_____

_____

_____

_____

_____

_____

_____

_____

_____

9. Read Hebrews 12:1-2 Jesus is our example, how was He able to endure the cross?

_____

_____

_____

_____

_____

_____

_____

_____

Does understanding the example of Christ help you to more willingly endure your daily crosses with joy? Explain your answer.

_____

_____

_____

_____

_____

_____

_____

_____

_____

_____

List 3 specific goals for personal growth in the character quality of Joy…

1) _____

_____

_____

_____

_____

_____

2) _____

_____

_____

_____

_____

3) _____

_____

_____

_____

_____

_____

_____

Joy

Personal Notes on Joy

_____
_____
_____
_____
_____
_____
_____
_____
_____
_____
_____
_____
_____
_____
_____
_____
_____
_____
_____
_____
_____
_____
_____

Self Control

DEFINITION: Restraint exercised over one's own impulses, emotions, or desires.

Self-Control, or a lack of self-control, shows up in almost every area of our daily lives. Our commitment to self-control affects our eating habits, study habits, hygiene, propensity to anger, jealousy, envy, and so much more.

Not surprisingly, God's Word addresses this area of self-control in the believer's life. Let's look into scripture to understand God's standards of self-control.

1. Read Daniel 1:1-17. In verse 8, why did Daniel seek permission to abstain from the King's food?

_____

_____

_____

_____

_____

_____

_____

So often, self-control begins with the initial step of simply "making up our mind" to do what is appropriate.

_____

_____

_____

_____

_____

_____

Re-read verses 9 and 17. What did God provide as a blessing for practicing self-control?

_____

_____

_____

2. Read Proverbs 25:28. To what is a man with no self-control compared?

_____

_____

_____

What does this look like today?

_____

_____

_____

_____

3. In Acts 24:25, Paul links self-control with righteousness and the judgment to come, causing fear in the heart of Felix. How are these three concepts linked together in our daily lives?

_____

_____

_____

_____

_____

_____

_____

_____

_____

"By constant self-discipline and self-control you can develop greatness of character."
—Grenville Kleiser

Grenville Kleiser (1868-1935) was a North American author. Grenville Kleiser was born in 1868 in Toronto, Canada. He married Elizabeth Thompson in 1894. Grenville died in August, 1935 in New York City. He was the author of a long list of inspirational books and guides to oratorical success and personal development. Kleiser also worked as an instructor in Public Speaking at Yale Divinity School, Yale University.

React to the above quote. Do you agree or disagree?

_____

_____

_____

_____

_____

_____

_____

_____

4. Read I Corinthians 7:5. Who can become involved in our lives when we lack self-control?

_____

_____

_____

_____

_____

_____

_____

_____

_____

_____

_____

5. Compare Galatians 5:22-23 and II Timothy 3:1-5. Looking honestly at your life, which list of character qualities most accurately characterizes you? What needs to change?

_____

_____

_____

_____

_____

_____

_____

_____

6. In II Peter 1:5-7, we see a progressive list of maturing character qualities. Right in the middle of the list is self-control, sandwiched between knowledge and perseverance. Explain how knowledge can enable self-control and why the result should then be perseverance.

_____

_____

_____

_____

_____

_____

_____

_____

_____

_____

7. Unlike Daniel, Samson did not practice self-control. Read Judges 16:16-19. What did Samson's lack of self-control cost him?

_____

_____

_____

_____

_____

_____

_____

_____

_____

_____

8. Self-control is a character quality God desires for both men and women. Compare God's call to self-control in these passages and note whom exactly is called to be self-controlled. Remember, self-controlled can also be translated as temperate or sensible.

I Timothy 3:2_____

_____

_____

Titus1:8 _____

_____

_____

Titus 2:2_____

_____

_____

Titus 2:5 _____

_____

_____

Titus 2:6 _____

_____

_____

9. Finally, if there is any doubt about God's desire for believers to practice self-control, read and record what you learn from Titus 2:11-12. Here, self-controlled may also be translated as sensible.

_____

_____

"Confirm thy soul in self-control."
—George Washington

George Washington   (February 22, 1732 [February 11, 1731] – December 14, 1799) was the dominant military and political leader of the new United States of America from 1775–1797, leading the American victory over Britain in the American Revolutionary War as commander in chief of the Continental Army, 1775–1783, and presiding over the writing of the Constitution in 1787. As the unanimous choice to serve as the first president (1789–1797), he developed the forms and rituals of government that have been used ever since, and built a strong, well-financed national government that avoided war, suppressed rebellion and won acceptance among Americans of all types. Acclaimed ever since as the "Father of his country", Washington, along with Abraham Lincoln (1809–1865), has become a central icon of republican values, self sacrifice in the name of the nation, American nationalism and the ideal union of civic and military leadership.

List 3 specific goals for personal growth in the character quality of Self Control...

1) _____

_____

_____

_____

_____

_____

2) _____

_____

_____

_____

_____

3) _____

_____

_____

_____

_____

Personal Notes on Self Control

_____

_____

_____

_____

_____

_____

_____

_____

_____

_____

_____

_____

_____

_____

_____

_____

_____

_____

_____

_____

_____

_____

_____

_____

Compassion

DEFINITION: Sympathetic consciousness of others' distress together with a desire to alleviate it.

The character quality of compassion is not simply a feeling, such as pity or sympathy. Compassion takes those feelings and puts them into action.

Compassion is one of the character qualities that a child would describe as; "Jesus with skin on." While the non-Christian world can offer aid and relief, only followers of Christ can offer true life changing compassion.

1. When Saul and Jonathan were killed in battle, David's heartfelt desire was to show compassion to his beloved friend Jonathan's family. Read II Samuel 9 to see how David fulfilled this desire. Record your observations.

_____

_____

_____

_____

_____

2. Read Judges 2:18. Why did God show compassion to the Israelites? Explain your answer.

_____

_____

_____

_____

_____

_____

_____

_____

_____

Did they deserve that compassion? Yes or no?

_____

_____

_____

_____

_____

_____

_____

3. Read Romans 5:8. How did God demonstrate His compassion towards us? Write out your answer below....

_____

_____

_____

_____

_____

_____

_____

_____

_____

_____

Did we deserve that compassion?

_____

_____

_____

_____

_____

_____

_____

4. Although the world would disagree, scripture tells us that compassion, like respect, need not be earned.

Is there someone God is prompting you to show compassion toward? Write their name(s) below...

_____

_____

_____

_____

_____

_____

Have you been waiting to have them "earn" your compassion?

_____

_____

_____

**"Make no judgments where
you have no compassion"**
—Anne McGaffrey

Anne Inez McCaffrey (born 1 April 1926) is an author of science fiction and fantasy novels, best known for her *Dragonriders of Pern* series. Born in the United States, she is long-term resident of Ireland.

React to the quote by Ann McGafrey. Do you agree or disagree?

_____

_____

_____

_____

_____

_____

_____

_____

5. Read Psalms 103:13. What earthly picture does God's compassion towards us represent? Write out your answer.

_____

_____

_____

_____

_____

According to this verse, what does God require of us? Explain.

_____

_____

_____

_____

6. Christ is an exact representation of God the Father and we are to be like Christ. Record what Psalm 116:5 tells us that our God looks like.

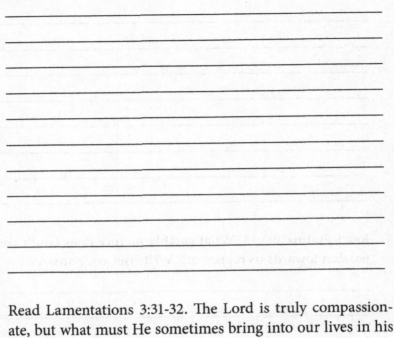

_____

_____

_____

_____

_____

_____

_____

_____

_____

7. Read Lamentations 3:31-32. The Lord is truly compassionate, but what must He sometimes bring into our lives in his compassion?

_____

_____

_____

_____

_____

_____

_____

8. What are the three qualities that God commands us to dispense to each other in Zechariah 7:9? List them below.

_____

_____

_____

_____

_____

_____

_____

9. Compassion does not come naturally to everyone, but as those chosen of God, we are told to put on a specific list of qualities. Read Colossians 3:12 to find out God's desire for character in our lives. Record what you learn.

_____

_____

_____

_____

_____

_____

_____

_____

_____

"Clothe yourselves with compassion, kindness, humility, gentleness, and patience."

—Apostle Paul

Compassion

List 3 specific goals for personal growth in the character quality of Compassion…

1) _____
_____
_____
_____
_____
_____

2) _____
_____
_____
_____
_____
_____

3) _____
_____
_____
_____
_____
_____
_____

Personal Notes on Compassion

_____

_____

_____

_____

_____

_____

_____

_____

_____

_____

_____

_____

_____

_____

_____

_____

_____

_____

_____

_____

_____

_____

Contentment

DEFINITION: The quality of being satisfied, feeling or manifesting satisfaction with one's possession, status, or situation.

While the world continually seeks for more, more, more, the mark of a Christian is their satisfaction with and thankfulness for all that God has provided. Let's allow scripture, not the world to shape our contentment.

1. In Philippians 4:11, Paul sets the standard for contentment in the believer's life. Read the verse and record what Paul says.

_____

_____

_____

_____

_____

_____

_____

_____

_____

_____

2. Philippians 4:12. further expands the definition of contentment for us. Restate this verse in your own words.

_____

_____

_____

_____

_____

_____

_____

_____

3. In Proverbs 19:23 we read what leads to a satisfied [contented]
sleep. What is needed to attain this satisfaction? Write out
your answer.

_____

_____

_____

_____

_____

_____

_____

_____

_____

_____

" True humility is contentment."
—Henri Frederic Amiel

Henri Frédéric Amiel (born 28 September 1821 – 11 May 1881) was a Swiss philosopher, poet and critic.

React to this quote. Do you agree or disagree?

_____

_____

_____

_____

_____

4. Read I Timothy 6:6. What must accompany godliness to achieve great gain? Explain your answer.

_____

_____

_____

_____

_____

5. Read Hebrews 13:5. Why can we be content with what we have? Write out your answer below.

_____

_____

_____

_____

_____

_____

_____

_____

6. The opposite of contentment is greed. Read Acts 5:1-5. Ananias wasn't simply greedy for money; he also wanted a reputation for giving more than he actually gave. How did God deal with his greed?

_____

_____

_____

_____

_____

_____

_____

_____

7. Read Ecclesiastes 4:8. What was considered as vanity and a grievous task?

_____

_____

_____

_____

_____

_____

_____

_____

8. Read I Timothy 6:7-8. With what are we to be content?

_____

_____

_____

_____

_____

_____

_____

_____

_____

_____

" True contentment is a thing as active as
agriculture. It is the power of getting out of
any situation all that there is in it.
It is arduous and it is rare."

—G.K. Chesterton

Gilbert Keith Chesterton (born 29 May 1874 – 14
June 1936) was an English writer. His prolific and diverse
output included philosophy, ontology, poetry, play writing, journalism, public lecturing and debating, biography,
Christian apologetics, fantasy and detective fiction.

Contentment

List 3 specific goals for personal growth in the character quality of Contentment...

1) _____

_____

_____

_____

_____

_____

2) _____

_____

_____

_____

_____

_____

3) _____

_____

_____

_____

_____

_____

_____

Personal Notes on Contentment

_____

_____

_____

_____

_____

_____

_____

_____

_____

_____

_____

_____

_____

_____

_____

_____

_____

_____

_____

_____

_____

_____

For Those Who Desire to Go Deeper

Below are extra verses to look up, study, and meditate upon. Remember, simply "learning" more verses won't change your behavior, thought processes, or attitude. Rather, it is as you incorporate the character qualities into your daily habits that change will occur, growth will be sustained, and Christ will be glorified. With each scripture reference, record what you learn from the text in the space provided. We've suggested a verse to memorize in conjunction with each character quality, but trust me; you can never memorize too much scripture, so feel free to memorize more than one!

INTEGRITY

Extra verses for study:

Psalm 15:1-3 _____

_____

_____

_____

Proverbs 28:6 _____

_____

_____

_____

Proverbs 19:1 _____

_____

_____

_____

Proverbs 20:7 _____

_____

_____

_____

I Peter 3:16 _____

_____

_____

_____

Luke 16:10 _____

_____

_____

_____

To memorize:

Proverbs 10:9 _____

_____

_____

_____

DILIGENCE

Extra verses for study:

Proverbs 21:5 _____

_____

_____

_____

I Kings 11:28 _____

_____

_____

_____

Ezra 7:23 _____

_____

_____

_____

Proverbs 12:14 _____

_____

_____

_____

I Timothy 5:17 _____

_____

_____

_____

Romans 12:8 _____

_____

_____

_____

To memorize:

Proverbs 12:14 _____

_____

_____

_____

_____

HONESTY

Extra verses for study:

Proverbs 12:22 _____

_____

_____

Proverbs 19:1 _____

_____

_____

I Peter 3:10-12 _____

_____

_____

Colossians 3:9 _____

_____

_____

Proverbs 16:13 _____

_____

_____

_____

Isaiah 33:15 _____

_____

_____

_____

To memorize:

Proverbs 12:22 _____

_____

_____

_____

_____

RESPECT

Extra verses for study:

Matthew 7:12 _____

_____

_____

_____

Romans 12:10 _____

_____

Philippians 2:3 _____

_____

_____

_____

I Samuel 2:30 _____

_____

_____

_____

I Thessalonians 5:12-13 _____

_____

_____

_____

Luke 6:31 _____

_____

_____

_____

To memorize:

Philippians 2:3 _____

_____

_____

_____

_____

_____

THANKFULNESS

Extra verses for study:

Psalm 107:1 _____

_____

_____

_____

Ephesians 5:20 _____

_____

_____

_____

Colossians 3:15-17 _____

_____

_____

_____

Colossians 4:2 _____

_____

_____

_____

Psalm 30:12 _____

_____

_____

_____

Psalm 100:4 _____

_____

_____

To memorize:

Psalm 100:4 _____

_____

_____

_____

_____

GENEROSITY

Extra verses for study:

Acts 20:35 _____

_____

_____

Luke 6:38 _____

_____

_____

I John 3:17 _____

_____

_____

Proverbs 19:17 _____

_____

_____

Deuteronomy 15:7-8 _____

_____

_____

_____

Psalm 112:5 _____

_____

_____

_____

To memorize:

Luke 6:38 _____

_____

_____

_____

_____

PATIENCE

Extra verses for study:

Romans 12:12 _____

_____

_____

Romans 8:25 _____

_____

_____

Galatians 6:9 _____

_____

_____

_____

Psalm 37:7-9_____

_____

_____

_____

I Corinthians 13:4 _____

_____

_____

_____

II Timothy 2:24 _____

_____

_____

_____

To memorize:

Galatians 6:9 _____

_____

_____

_____

_____

_____

RESPONSIBILITY

Extra verses for study:

Galatians 6:5 _____

_____

_____

_____

I Timothy 5:8 _____

_____

_____

_____

Romans 12:6-8 _____

_____

_____

_____

Luke 16:10 _____

_____

_____

_____

I Samuel 15:22 _____

_____

_____

_____

I Timothy 4:12 _____

_____

_____

To memorize:

Galatians 6:5 _____

_____

_____

_____

_____

JOY

Extra verses for study:

James 1:2 _____

_____

_____

Romans 15:13 _____

_____

_____

I Peter 4:8 _____

_____

_____

Proverbs 17:22 _____

_____

_____

James 1:2-4 _____

_____

_____

_____

Proverbs 10:28 _____

_____

_____

_____

To memorize:

James 1:2-4 _____

_____

_____

_____

_____

SELF-CONTROL

Extra verses for study:

I Corinthians 10:13 _____

_____

_____

I Corinthians 9:24-27 _____

_____

_____

Proverbs 16:32 _____

_____

_____

_____

II Timothy 1:7 _____

_____

_____

_____

I Corinthians 6:19 _____

_____

_____

_____

I Timothy 4:7 _____

_____

_____

_____

To memorize:

II Timothy 1:7 _____

_____

_____

_____

_____

_____

COMPASSION

Extra verses for study:

Ephesians 4:32 _____

_____

_____

_____

Mark 6:34 _____

_____

_____

_____

Galatians 6:2 _____

_____

_____

_____

James 1:27 _____

_____

_____

_____

Psalm 86:15 _____

_____

_____

_____

Psalm 41:1-2 _____

_____

_____

_____

To memorize:

Ephesians 4:32 _____

_____

_____

_____

_____

CONTENTMENT

Extra verses for study:

Luke 12:15 _____

_____

_____

_____

Philippians 4:19 _____

_____

_____

_____

I Corinthians 7:17 _____

_____

_____

_____

II Corinthians 12:10 _____

_____

_____

For Going Deeper

Proverbs 30:8-9 _____

_____

_____

_____

Proverbs 16:8 _____

_____

_____

_____

To memorize:

Philippians 4:19 _____

_____

_____

_____

_____

CONTACT US

Steve and Megan travel extensively facilitating parenting, marriage, and men's and women's conferences for churches and other organizations.

CONFERENCES AVAILABLE INCLUDE:

Parenting Matters
Marriage Matters
Character Matters
Second Mile Leadership for Men
When God Writes Your Story
The Wise Wife
The A-Z of a Character Healthy Homeschool
The Discipling Mom
The Toddler Toolbox and more....

To speak with Steve or Megan please call:
1-877-577-2736

Or send them an email by clicking the Contact Us tab at:
Characterhealth.com

also, follow them on twitter:
@SteveScheibner
@Meganscheibner
@CharacterHealth

Or check out Steve and Megan's Blogs at:
SteveScheibner.com
MeganScheibner.com

OTHER BOOKS BY MEGAN ANN SCHEIBNER:

In My Seat:
A Pilot's Story from Sept. 10th–11th

Grand Slam:
An Athletes Guide to Success in Life

Rise and Shine:
Recipes and Routines For Your Morning

Lunch and Literature

Dinner and Discipleship

Studies in Character

**The King of Thing and the Kingdom
of Thingdom**

**An A to Z Guide For Characterhealthy
Homeschooling**

OTHER BOOKS BY STEVE SCHEIBNER:

Bible Basics

(Now available with a DVD for small group studies)

BOOKS BY STEVE AND MEGAN SCHEIBNER:

Eight Rules of Communication For Successful Marriages

Studies in Character

The King of Thing and the Kingdom of Thingdom

DVD Series Available:

Parenting Matters:
The Nine Practices of the Pro-Active Parent

Character Matters:
The Nine Practices of Character
Healthy Youth

The Toddler Toolbox

Battling With Behavior

Bible Basics

Grandparenting With Purpose

You can find these books and other resources at:
CharacterHealth.com

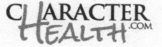

All biographies are from Wikipedia
the online encyclopedia.

All Bible references are from the
New American Standard Bible.